GOUT DIET COOKBOOK FOR SENIORS

Delicious and Simple Low-Purine Recipes to Manage Flares.

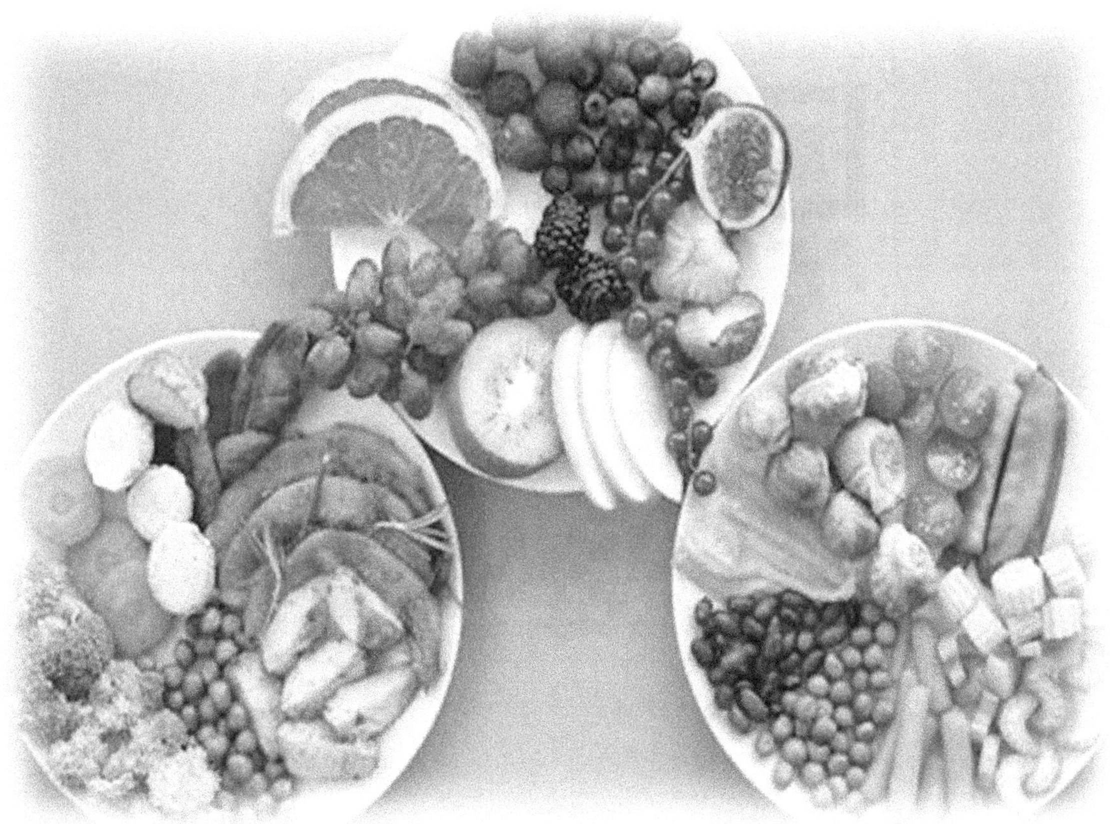

CHRISTIANA WHITE

GAIN ACCESS TO MORE BOOKS

DISCLAIMER

The recipes in this cookbook are provided for informational purposes only and are not intended as medical or professional advice. While the author and publisher have made every effort to ensure the accuracy and effectiveness of the recipes, they are not responsible for any adverse effects r consequences resulting from the use of the suggestions herein.

The information in this cookbook should not replace professional advice. Readers are advised to consult a healthcare provider or a culinary professional before making any significant changes to their diet or cooking practices.

Nutritional information is approximate and should be used as a guide only. Variations may occur due to product availability, food preparation, portion size, and other factors.

The author and publisher disclaim any liability in connection with the use of this information. It is the reader's responsibility to determine the value and quality of any recipe or instructions provided for food preparation and to determine the nutritional adequacy of the food to be consumed.

ABOUT THE AUTHOR

When it comes to tasty and nutritious cookbooks that turn wellness into a delightful journey, Christiana White is the author you turn to. She approaches cooking from a new angle and has a passion for creating wholesome food.

Motivated by her own pursuit of health, Christiana's books on Amazon are brimming with delectable recipes that demonstrate that eating healthily can be both simple and enjoyable. Her creative method makes cooking approachable to all skill levels by fusing entire, simple foods with flavors from around the world.

Readers of Christiana's meals gush about the beneficial effects her foods have on their lives outside of the kitchen. Her books are more than just recipes; they're guides for a happier, better way of life, resulting in everything from more energy to a revitalized passion for cooking.

Come along with Christiana to discover how to turn your meals into satisfying and joyful experiences. Discover the delightful intersection of health and flavor by delving into the colourful world of her cookbooks.

TABLE OF CONTENTS.

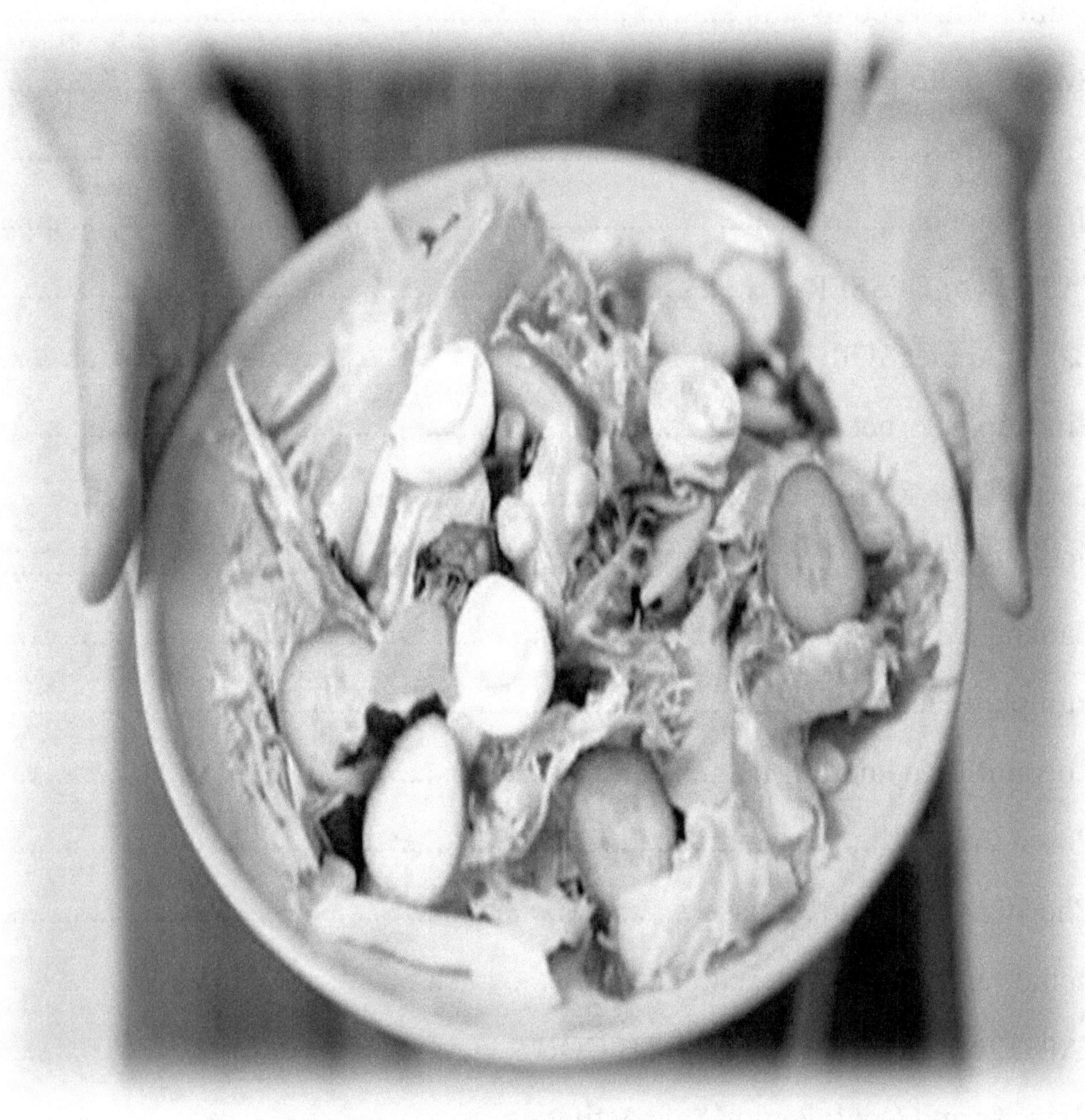

INTRODUCTION

With our Cookbook, you can discover the secret to joyful eating and gout management!

Consider a world in which every meal is a celebration, a symphony of tastes that dances on your palate while nourishing your body. This is what the "Gout Diet Cookbook for Seniors" promises to elders everywhere.

Gout is commonly associated with pain and dietary restrictions. But what if I told you that managing gout does not entail giving up your favorite foods? Our cookbook exemplifies this very attitude. It's more than simply a compilation of recipes; it's a gateway to a flavour-filled existence free of gout flare-ups.

Seniors around the world have adopted this cookbook as their culinary bible, improving their diets and lifestyles. They've discovered the thrill of cooking with products that are as gentle on their joints as they are on their palates. They have discovered that a gout-friendly diet can be both enjoyable and nutritious, and they are thriving!

From the rustic appeal of our Sunny Citrus Parfait to the cozy embrace of our Vegetable Lasagna, each meal celebrates life after gout. These recipes have not only delighted palates, but have also rekindled the joy of cooking and eating for many seniors who felt their days of good food had passed.

So, come to our kitchen, where health meets taste, and let us take you on a culinary adventure that will revolutionize the way you think about the gout diet. This is more than a cookbook; it's a new chapter in your life, full of delectable possibilities and pain-free days.

Welcome to the "Gout Diet Cookbook for Seniors," where each recipe represents a step toward a happier, healthier you.

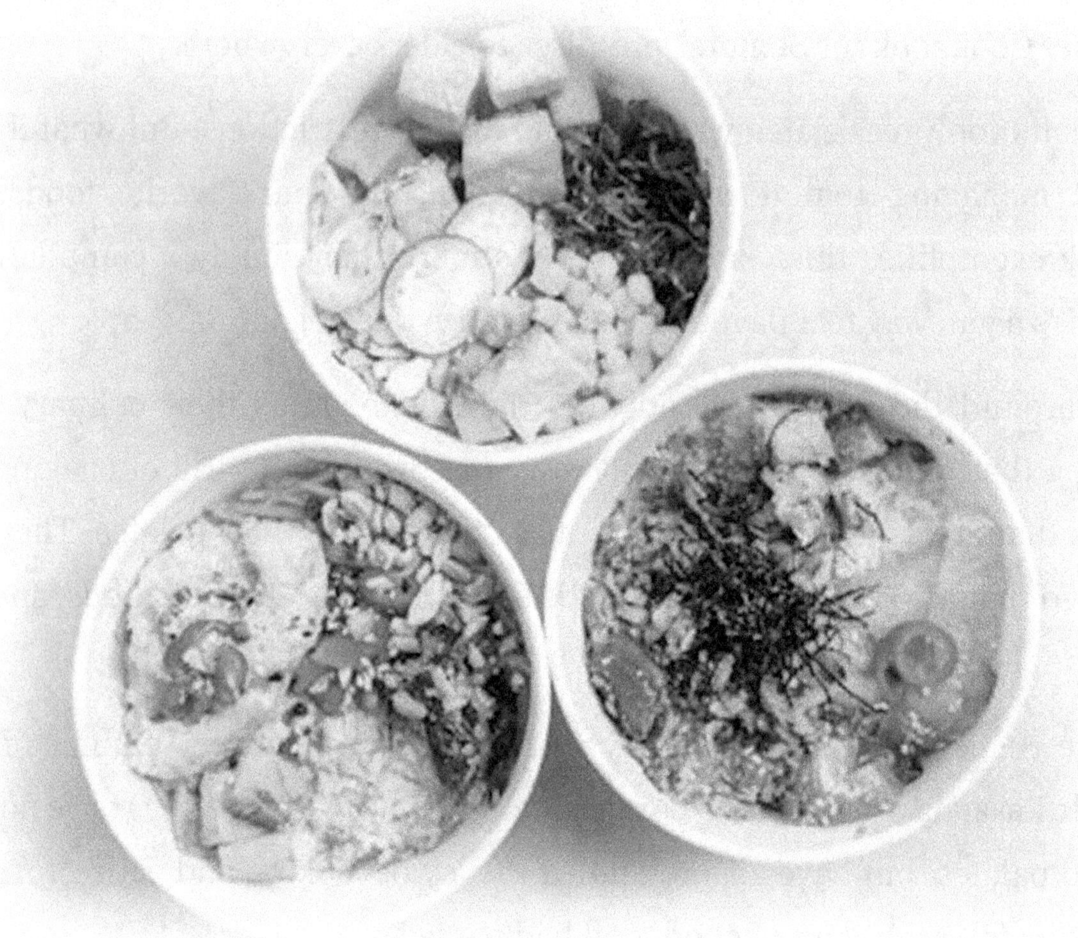

CHAPTER 1: UNDERSTANDING GOUT.

Gout and Ageing

Gout is a kind of inflammatory arthritis that causes sudden, intense outbreaks of pain, swelling, redness, and tenderness in the joints, usually near the base of the big toe.

As we age, our bodies go through a variety of physiological changes that raise our chances of acquiring gout. Gout management is especially crucial for elderly, as it can have a substantial impact on their quality of life and mobility.

Increased Prevalence with Age.

Gout is the most frequent type of inflammatory arthritis among the elderly. Epidemiological studies have revealed that the incidence and prevalence of gout increase with age in both sexes. This increase is attributable in part to greater life expectancy in industrialized countries, which exposes people to age-related disorders such as hypertension and metabolic syndrome, both of which are linked to an increased risk of gout.

Physiological Changes

The kidney's ability to operate reduces with age, resulting in less efficient uric acid clearance, which, at high levels, can cause gout. Furthermore, seniors frequently have other comorbidities, such as cardiovascular disease and diabetes, which complicates gout treatment.

Medication Management

Older persons are more prone to take several drugs, which can interfere with gout therapy or potentially lead to high uric acid levels. To avoid side effects and interactions, drugs must be managed carefully.

Dietary Considerations

A rigorous gout diet is essential for elders. This diet limits meals high in purines, which can raise uric acid levels. Avoid foods such as red meat, organ meats, certain seafood, sugary beverages, and excessive alcohol.

Instead, seniors should consume low-fat dairy products, whole grains, plant oils, vegetables, some fruits, vitamin C supplements, and coffee, all of which have been shown to help lower uric acid levels.

Lifestyle Modifications

Staying hydrated by consuming plenty of water, maintaining a healthy weight, and avoiding sweetened beverages and alcohol can all help prevent gout episodes. Low-impact activities are also useful to overall health and can aid with weight management.

Complications

If left untreated, gout can progress to more serious illnesses like chronic gouty arthritis and the formation of tophi, which are painful masses of uric acid crystals that can grow in joints and other tissues. Recurrent gout attacks can damage joints over time, and uric acid crystals accumulated in the kidneys can lead to kidney stones.

Prevention and Treatment

Lifestyle adjustments, such as diet and weight management, are examples of preventive interventions. Gout attacks may be treated with nonsteroidal anti-inflammatory medications (NSAIDs), corticosteroids, or colchicine. Long-term therapy may involve prescribing uric acid-lowering drugs such as allopurinol or febuxostat.

Gout can have a substantial impact on elders, but with correct therapy, which includes medication, nutrition, and lifestyle changes, gout symptoms can be controlled and the risk of complications reduced. Seniors and their caregivers must work together with healthcare experts to develop a gout management strategy that takes into account the unique problems of aging.

The Science of Uric Acid

Understanding uric acid and its relationship to our food is critical to controlling gout and living a healthy, active lifestyle.

What is uric acid?

Uric acid is a natural waste product produced when your body breaks down compounds known as purines. Normally, uric acid dissolves in your blood and is expelled by your kidney. However, if you have too much uric acid or your kidneys are unable to clear it adequately, the excess can form crystals that accumulate in your joints, causing gout symptoms.

Purines are the building blocks of uric acid.

Many of the foods we eat include purines. Some foods are naturally high in purines, while others help to produce uric acid in different ways. Here's what you should know.

- Foods high in purine include organ meats (liver, kidney, sweetbreads), shellfish (anchovies, sardines, mussels), red meat, and alcohol (particularly beer).
- Foods with Moderate Purine Content: These include some fish (tuna, trout), poultry, and legumes.
- Low-Purine Foods: This category includes most fruits and vegetables, whole grains, low-fat dairy products, eggs, and nuts.

While managing gout can be difficult, realize that you're not alone. By following a gout diet, staying hydrated, and working with your doctor, you can successfully regulate your uric acid levels and live a more pleasant and active lifestyle.

CHAPTER 2: DIETARY FOUNDATIONS

The Gout Diet Basics

Adopting a low-purine diet is an important technique for treating gout, particularly in seniors. This diet focuses on minimizing purine-rich meals, which are converted into uric acid, a chemical that can accumulate in joints and induce gout attacks.

Understand the Purine Levels in Foods

- Avoid or limit meals high in purine, such as red meats, organ meats, and certain shellfish like anchovies, sardines, mussels, scallops, trout, and tuna.
- Moderate Purine Foods: Consume in moderation. This includes poultry, legumes (e.g., beans and lentils), mushrooms, spinach, and asparagus.
- Low-purine foods are encouraged in the diet. These include eggs, nuts, low-fat dairy products, bread and cereals (not whole grain), pasta, noodles, fruits, and the majority of vegetables.

Concentrate on hydration.

- Drink plenty of water throughout the day to help flush uric acid out of your system.

Limit your alcohol intake.

- Alcohol, particularly beer, can enhance purine production and should be avoided or ingested in small doses.

Maintain a healthy weight.

- Excess weight can raise uric acid levels. Aim for moderate weight loss by eating a balanced diet and engaging in regular physical activity.

Select the Right Carbohydrates.

- Choose complex carbs such as fruits, vegetables, and whole grains. Avoid sugary foods and beverages, particularly those made with high-fructose corn syrup.

Include low-fat dairy products.

- Low-fat milk and yogurt have been linked to reduce uric acid levels and are suggested as part of a gout-friendly diet.

Consume Healthy Fats

- Use plant-based oils in your cooking and salads. Limit the saturated fats found in butter and fatty cuts of meat.

Be mindful of portion sizes.

- Even when eating low-purine foods, portion control is essential to avoid consuming too many calories.

Consider the DASH Diet Approach.

- The DASH diet, which emphasizes fruits, vegetables, whole grains, and low-fat dairy, is similar to a low-purine diet and may benefit persons with gout.

Regular Checkups

- Check your uric acid levels on a regular basis with your doctor to confirm that your diet is adequately treating your gout.

Following these strategies can help seniors with gout manage their symptoms and lessen the frequency of gout attacks.

As we age, our nutritional needs change, making it even more crucial to fuel our bodies with the proper nutrients to sustain health, energy, and vitality. However, healthy eating does not have to imply losing flavour.

With a little imagination and understanding, seniors may consume delightful meals that also feed their bodies.

Key Nutrients for Seniors

- Protein is essential for maintaining muscular mass, strength, and immunological function. Good sources include lean meats, chicken, fish, beans, lentils, eggs, and dairy products.
- Calcium is essential for bone health and osteoporosis prevention. It can be found in milk, leafy green vegetables, fortified cereals, and tofu.
- Vitamin D: Aids calcium absorption and promotes immunological function. Sunlight, fatty fish, egg yolks, and fortified foods are excellent sources.
- Fiber: Improves digestive health and can help regulate cholesterol and blood sugar levels. Concentrate on whole grains, fruits, veggies, legumes, and lentils.
- Potassium is essential for heart health and blood pressure regulation. Bananas, potatoes, sweet potatoes, legumes, and leafy greens are high in potassium.
- B vitamins promote energy production and neuronal function. Found in whole grains, meat, fish, eggs, and leafy green vegetables.

- Omega-3 Fatty Acids: They promote heart health and may reduce inflammation. You can get them from fatty fish (salmon, tuna, mackerel), flaxseeds, chia seeds, and walnuts.

Tips to Balance Health and Flavor

- Experiment with Spices and Herbs: Instead of using salt and sugar, add flavour to your cuisine with herbs and spices. Experiment with various cuisines and flavour combinations.
- Prioritize Freshness: Select fresh, seasonal fruits and vegetables for the best flavour and nutrient value.
- Cook at Home: Cooking at home allows you to manage the ingredients and experiment with healthier cooking methods such as grilling, baking, or steaming.
- Eat Mindfully: Pay attention to hunger and fullness cues, and enjoy the tastes of your meal.

Healthy eating is a journey rather than a goal. You can enjoy great meals that nourish both your body and spirit by focusing on nutrient-dense foods, experimenting with new Flavors, and cooking at home.

Sunny Citrus Parfait.

- **Serves: 1**
- **Prep time: 10 minutes.**

Ingredients:

- 1/2 cup of low-fat Greek yogurt
- One orange, peeled and sectioned
- 1/2 grapefruit, peeled and sectioned.
- One spoonful of honey.
- Two tablespoons of granola (no high-purine nuts).

Instructions:

- In a glass, layer half the Greek yogurt.
- Add a layer of orange and grapefruit segments.
- Drizzle with half the honey.
- Sprinkle with a tablespoon of granola.
- Continue layering with the remaining ingredients.
- Serve immediately and enjoy!

Nutritional Information: 250 calories, 3g fat, 47g carbs, 13g protein, and low purines.

<u>Cherry Oatmeal Delight</u>

- **Serves: 1**
- **Prep time: 5 minutes.**
- **Cook time: 15 minutes.**

Ingredients:

- 1/2 cup rolled oats.
- 1 cup water or low-fat milk.
- 1/2 cup fresh cherries, pitted and halved.
- One-quarter teaspoon cinnamon
- 1 tablespoon of almond slivers.

Instructions:

- In a small saucepan, heat the water or milk until it boils.
- Add the oats and decrease the heat to a simmer.
- Cook for 10-15 minutes, stirring regularly, until the oats have softened.
- Mix in cinnamon and half of the cherries.
- Transfer the oats to a bowl and top with the remaining cherries and almond slivers.
- Serve warm and enjoy the Flavors.

Nutritional Information: calories: 220, fat: 4g, carbohydrates: 40g, protein: 6g, purines: low.

<u>Egg White Vegetable Scramble</u>

- **Serves: 1**
- **Prep time: 5 minutes.**
- **Cooking Time: 10 minutes.**

Ingredients:

- Three egg whites.
- 1/2 cup chopped bell peppers.
- 1/4 cup diced onions
- One-quarter cup chopped tomatoes
- Add salt and pepper to taste.
- One teaspoon of olive oil.

Instructions:

- Heat olive oil in a nonstick skillet over medium heat.
- Sauté the onions and bell peppers until tender.
- Stir in the tomatoes and simmer for another 2 minutes.
- Pour in the egg whites and scramble until completely done.
- Season with salt and pepper.
- Serve hot and enjoy a bright start to the day.

Nutritional Information: calories: 120, fat: 3g, carbs: 8g, protein: 14g, purines: low.

Almond Butter Toast

- **Serves: 1**
- **Prep time: 5 minutes.**
- **Cook time: two minutes.**

Ingredients:

- One slice of whole grain bread.
- Two tablespoons of almond butter.
- 1/2 banana, sliced
- 1/4 teaspoon ground flaxseed.

Instructions:

- Toast the whole grain bread to your preference.
- Spread the almond butter evenly on the toast.
- Garnish with banana slices and ground flaxseed.
- Serve immediately for a crunchy, creamy breakfast.

Nutritional Information: calories: 280, fat: 16g, carbs: 30g, protein: 10g, purines: low

<u>Berry Banana Smoothie</u>

- **Serves: 1**
- **Prep time: 5 minutes.**

Ingredients:

- One-half banana.
- half cup mixed berries (strawberries, blueberries, raspberries)
- 1/2 cup of low-fat Greek yogurt
- Half-cup water or almond milk
- One teaspoon of honey (optional)

Instructions:

- Place all items in a blender.
- Blend until smooth and creamy.
- Pour into a glass and enjoy your pleasant and nutritious smoothie.

Nutritional Information: calories: 180, fat: 1g, carbs: 36g, protein: 10g, purines: low.

<u>Apple Cinnamon Porridge</u>

- **Serves: 1**
- **Prep time: 5 minutes.**
- **Cook time: 15 minutes.**

Ingredients:

- 1/2 cup rolled oats.
- 1 cup water or low-fat milk.
- One apple, peeled and diced
- 1/2 teaspoon of ground cinnamon.
- One teaspoon of honey (optional)

Instructions:

- Heat water or milk in a pot until it boils.
- Add the oats and diced apple, then decrease the heat to low.
- Add cinnamon and cook for 10-15 minutes until the oats are tender.
- Add honey if desired.
- Serve warm.

Nutritional Information: calories: 215, fat: 2.5g, carbs: 43g, protein: 5g, purines: low.

<u>Tomato Basil Omelet</u>

- **Serves: 1**
- **Prep time: 5 minutes.**
- **Cook for 5 minutes.**

Ingredients:

- Two egg whites.
- One small tomato, chopped
- Two finely chopped basil leaves.
- Add salt and pepper to taste.
- One teaspoon of olive oil.

Instructions:

- Mix the egg whites with salt and pepper.
- Heat the olive oil in a skillet over medium heat.
- Pour in egg whites and simmer for 1 minute.
- Add the diced tomato and basil over top.
- Fold the omelette and cook until it's set.
- Serve hot.

Nutritional Information: 110 calories, 5g fat, 4g carbs, 11g protein, low purines.

<u>Avocado Egg Salad.</u>

- **Servings: two.**
- **Prep time: 10 minutes.**

Ingredients:

- Four hardboiled egg whites, chopped
- One ripe avocado, mashed
- One tablespoon of lemon juice.
- Add salt and pepper to taste.
- Wholegrain bread for serving.

Instructions:

- In a bowl, combine egg whites and avocado.
- Combine lemon juice, salt, and pepper.
- Mix until thoroughly blended.
- Serve on whole-grain toast or with salad.

Nutritional Information: 220 calories, 15g fat, 10g carbs, 12g protein, and low purines.

<u>Peachy Keen Muesli.</u>

- **Serves: 1**
- **Prep time: 5 minutes.**

Ingredients:

- 1/2 cup rolled oats.
- Half-cup low-fat yogurt
- One peach, diced
- One spoonful of honey.
- One tablespoon of slivered almonds

Instructions:

- In a bowl, combine the oats and yogurt.
- Garnish with diced peach and almond.
- Drizzle with honey.
- Serve immediately or leave overnight.

Nutritional Information: calories: 285, fat: 4g, carbs: 53g, protein: 10g, purines: low.

<u>Spinach and Feta Wrap</u>

- **Serves: 1**
- **Prep time: 10 minutes.**
- **Cook for 5 minutes.**

Ingredients:

- One whole grain tortilla.
- 1/2 cup of spinach leaves.
- 1/4 cup crumbled feta cheese.
- One egg white.
- Add salt and pepper to taste.
- One teaspoon of olive oil.

Instructions:

- Cook the egg whites in olive oil and season with salt and pepper.
- Heat the tortilla in a dry pan.
- Put spinach leaves on the tortilla.
- Combine the scrambled egg and feta cheese.
- Roll up the tortillas and serve warm.

Nutritional Information: 180 calories, 9g fat, 16g carbs, 11g protein, low purines.

<u>**Quinoa Tabbouleh.**</u>

- **Servings: two.**
- **Prep time: 15 minutes.**
- **Cook time: 15 minutes.**

Ingredients:

- One cup cooked quinoa.
- 1 cup chopped fresh parsley.
- 1/2 cup of chopped fresh mint.
- 1/2 cup of diced cucumber.
- 1/2 cup of diced tomatoes.
- Two teaspoons of olive oil.
- Juice from 1 lemon
- Add salt and pepper to taste.

Instructions:

- Cook the quinoa according to the package directions and let it cool.
- In a large bowl, combine the chilled quinoa, parsley, mint, cucumber, and tomatoes.
- In a small bowl, combine olive oil, lemon juice, salt, and pepper.
- Toss the dressing into the quinoa mixture.
- Refrigerate for at least 30 minutes prior to serving.

Nutritional Information: 310 calories, 14g fat, 42g carbs, 8g protein, low purines.

<u>Grilled Chicken Salad.</u>

- **Servings: two.**
- **Prep time: 10 minutes.**
- **Cooking Time: 10 minutes.**

Ingredients:

- Two boneless, skinless chicken breasts (4 ounces each)
- Four cups mixed salad greens.
- 1/2 cup cherry tomatoes, cut in half
- 1/4 cup of sliced red onion.
- Two tablespoons of balsamic vinaigrette

Instructions:

- Grill the chicken breasts over medium heat until fully done.
- Let the chicken rest for a few minutes before slicing.
- Combine the salad greens, cherry tomatoes, and red onion in a large bowl.
- Add sliced chicken and drizzle with balsamic vinaigrette.
- Serve immediately.

Nutritional Information: 275 calories, 9g fat, 10g carbs, 35g protein, moderate purines.

<u>Lentil Soup with Vegetables</u>

- **Servings: four.**
- **Prep time: 10 minutes.**
- **Cooking Time: 40 minutes.**

Ingredients:

- 1 cup of dried lentils, washed
- One tablespoon of olive oil.
- 1 onion, chopped
- Two carrots, chopped
- Two celery stalks, diced
- Four cups of veggie broth.
- One teaspoon dried thyme.
- Add salt and pepper to taste.

Instructions:

- Heat the olive oil in a big pot over medium heat.
- Cook the onion, carrots, and celery until softened.
- Combine the lentils, vegetable broth, and thyme.
- Bring to a boil, then reduce the heat and simmer for 30 minutes.
- Season with salt and pepper.
- Serve hot.

Nutritional Information: 240 calories, 4g fat, 38g carbs, 14g protein, and low purines.

<u>Turkey and Avocado Wrap</u>

- **Serves: 1**
- **Prep time: 5 minutes.**

Ingredients:

- One whole grain tortilla.
- Four ounces of sliced turkey breast
- 1/2 ripe avocado sliced
- 1/2 cup of spinach leaves.
- One tablespoon mustard.

Instructions:

- Place the tortilla flat on a dish.
- Spread mustard on the tortilla.
- Place the turkey, avocado slices, and spinach over top.
- Roll the tortilla tightly and cut in half.
- Serve immediately or wrap as a to-go lunch.

Nutritional Information: 370 calories, 16g fat, 36g carbs, 22g protein, low purines.

<u>Cucumber Sandwiches.</u>

- **Servings: two.**
- **Prep time: 5 minutes.**

Ingredients:

- Four pieces of whole grain bread.
- 1/2 cucumber, thinly sliced
- 2 tablespoons softened cream cheese.
- Dill or chives as garnish.

Instructions:

- Spread the cream cheese equally on the slices of bread.
- Arrange cucumber slices on two slices of bread.
- Season with dill or chives.
- Top with the remaining bread slices.
- Cut in quarters and serve.

Nutritional Information: 180 calories, 6g fat, 26g carbs, 6g protein, low purines.

<u>**Carrot and Ginger Puree**</u>

- **Servings: two.**
- **Prep time: 10 minutes.**
- **Cook time: 20 minutes.**

Ingredients:

- 4 big peeled and sliced carrots.
- One tablespoon of grated fresh ginger.
- Two cups of veggie broth.
- Add salt and pepper to taste.

Instructions:

- In a pot, heat the vegetable broth until it boils.
- Add carrots and ginger, then decrease heat to a simmer.
- Cook until carrots are soft, about 20 minutes.
- Use an immersion blender to smooth up the mixture.
- Add salt and pepper to taste.
- Serve warm.

Nutritional Information: 95 calories, 0.5g fat, 22g carbs, 2g protein, and low purines.

<u>Tofu Stir-Fry</u>

- **Servings: two.**
- **Prep time: 15 minutes.**
- **Cooking Time: 10 minutes.**

Ingredients:

- One block of firm tofu, drained and cubed
- Two cups of mixed vegetables (bell peppers, broccoli, carrots).
- One tablespoon of soy sauce.
- One teaspoon of sesame oil.
- One garlic clove, minced

Instructions:

- Heat the sesame oil in a pan over medium heat.
- Add the garlic and sauté until fragrant.
- Increase the heat to high, then add the tofu and vegetables.
- Stir-fry for 5-7 minutes, or until the vegetables are soft and crunchy.
- Drizzle with soy sauce and toss until evenly coated.
- Serve hot.

Nutritional Information: 150 calories, 9g fat, 8g carbs, 12g protein, low purines.

<u>Mediterranean Chickpea Salad</u>

- **Servings: four.**
- **Prep time: 15 minutes.**

Ingredients:

- 1 can drained and rinsed chickpeas.
- One cucumber, diced
- 1 bell pepper, diced
- 1/4 cup coarsely chopped red onion.
- 1/4 cup crumbled feta cheese.
- Two teaspoons of olive oil.
- Juice from 1 lemon
- Add salt and pepper to taste.

Instructions:

- In a large mixing basin, add chickpeas, cucumber, bell pepper, and red onion.
- In a small bowl, combine olive oil, lemon juice, salt, and pepper.
- Pour dressing over salad and toss to mix.
- Garnish with feta cheese before serving.
- Serve cold or room temperature.

Nutritional Information: 250 calories, 10g fat, 30g carbs, 10g protein, low purines.

- **Servings: four.**
- **Prep time: 10 minutes.**
- **Cook for 30 minutes.**

Ingredients:

- 2 cups pumpkin puree.
- 1 onion, chopped
- Two cups of veggie broth.
- One cup low-fat milk.
- One teaspoon of cinnamon.
- Add salt and pepper to taste.

Instructions:

- In a pot, sauté the onion until transparent.
- Combine the pumpkin puree, vegetable broth, and cinnamon.
- Bring to a boil, then simmer for 20 minutes.
- Stir in the milk and heat thoroughly.
- Blend until smooth, if desired.
- Season with salt and pepper.
- Serve warm.

Nutritional Information: 90 calories, 2g fat, 16g carbs, 3g protein, low purines.

<u>Broccoli & Pine Nut Pasta</u>

- **Servings: two.**
- **Prep time: 5 minutes.**
- **Cook time: 15 minutes.**

Ingredients:

- Two cups of whole grain pasta.
- 1 cup of broccoli florets.
- Two tablespoons of pine nuts.
- One tablespoon of olive oil.
- One garlic clove, minced
- Add salt and pepper to taste.

Instructions:

- Cook the pasta according to package directions, then add the broccoli in the last three minutes.
- Drain the pasta and broccoli, reserving 1/4 cup boiling water.
- In the same saucepan, heat the olive oil over medium heat.
- Sauté garlic and pine nuts until golden.
- Return the pasta and broccoli to the pot and add the reserved water.
- Toss everything until fully combined.
- Season with salt and pepper.
- Serve warm.

Nutritional Information: 350 calories, 14g fat, 48g carbs, 12g protein, low purines.

<u>Baked Salmon and Dill</u>

- **Servings: two.**
- **Prep time: 5 minutes.**
- **Cook time: 15 minutes.**

Ingredients:

- Two salmon fillets, 4 ounces each.
- 1 tablespoon fresh dill, chopped
- One lemon, cut
- Add salt and pepper to taste.

Instructions:

- Preheat the oven to 375° F (190° C).
- Arrange the salmon fillets on a baking pan lined with parchment paper.
- Season with salt and pepper.
- Garnish each fillet with dill and lemon wedges.
- Bake for 15 minutes, or until the salmon flakes easily with a fork.

Nutritional Information: 240 calories, 14g fat, 0g carbs, 24g protein, moderate purines.

Stuffed Bell Peppers

- **Servings: four.**
- **Prep time: 20 minutes.**
- **Cook for 30 minutes.**

Ingredients:

- 4 bell peppers with tops removed and seeded
- One cup of cooked brown rice.
- Rinse and drain 1 cup canned black beans.
- One cup corn kernel.
- 1/2 cup of tomato sauce.
- One teaspoon cumin.
- Add salt and pepper to taste.

Instructions:

- Preheat the oven to 350°F (175° C).
- In a bowl, combine the brown rice, black beans, corn, tomato sauce, and cumin.
- Season with salt and pepper.
- Pack the mixture into the bell peppers.
- Arrange the filled peppers in a baking dish and cover with foil.
- Bake for 30 minutes, until the peppers are soft.

Nutritional Information: 200 calories, 1.5g fat, 40g carbs, 8g protein, low purines.

<u>Grilled Turkey Burgers.</u>

- **Servings: four.**
- **Prep time: 10 minutes.**
- **Cooking Time: 10 minutes.**

Ingredients:

- One pound ground turkey breast.
- One-quarter cup breadcrumbs
- One egg white.
- One tablespoon of Worcestershire sauce.
- Add salt and pepper to taste.

Instructions:

- Preheat the grill to medium-high heat.
- In a bowl, combine the ground turkey, breadcrumbs, egg white, and Worcestershire sauce.
- Season with salt and pepper.
- Form into four patties.
- Grill for 5 minutes per side, or until thoroughly done.

Nutritional Information: 180 calories, 2g fat, 5g carbs, 35g protein, moderate purines.

<u>Vegetable Lasagna</u>

- **Servings: six.**
- **Prep time: 30 minutes.**
- **Cook for 45 minutes.**

Ingredients:

- 9 lasagna noodles (cooked)
- Two cups of ricotta cheese
- 1 egg
- Two cups of chopped spinach.
- 1 zucchini, sliced
- Two cups marinara sauce.
- 1 cup shredded mozzarella cheese.

Instructions:

- Preheat the oven to 375° F (190° C).
- In a bowl, combine the ricotta cheese and egg.
- Spread a layer of marinara sauce on the bottom of a baking dish.
- Layer the noodles, ricotta mixture, spinach, zucchini, and sauce.
- Repeat layers, then top with mozzarella cheese.
- Cover with foil and bake for 45 minutes.
- Remove the lid and continue baking for an additional 15 minutes, or until the cheese is bubbling.

Nutritional Information: 350 calories, 10g fat, 45g carbs, 20g protein, low purines.

<u>Lemon Herb Chicken</u>

- **Servings: four.**
- **Prep time: 10 minutes.**
- **Cook time: 25 minutes.**

Ingredients:

- 4 chicken breasts, 4 ounces each.
- One lemon, juiced
- Two teaspoons of olive oil.
- 1 tablespoon mixed herbs (thyme, rosemary, and parsley).
- Add salt and pepper to taste.

Instructions:

- Preheat the oven to 375° F (190° C).
- In a bowl, combine the lemon juice, olive oil, and herbs.
- Season the chicken with salt and pepper.
- Put the chicken in a baking dish and pour the lemon herb mixture over it.
- Bake for 25 minutes, or until the chicken is cooked through.

Nutritional Information: 220 calories, 9g fat, 3g carbs, 30g protein, moderate purines.

<u>Roasted Eggplant and Quinoa</u>

- **Servings: two.**
- **Prep time: 10 minutes.**
- **Cook for 30 minutes.**

Ingredients:

- 1 large eggplant, cubed.
- One cup quinoa.
- Two cups of veggie broth.
- Two teaspoons of olive oil.
- One teaspoon of garlic powder.
- Add salt and pepper to taste.

Instructions:

- Preheat your oven to 400°F (200°C).
- Mix the eggplant cubes with olive oil, garlic powder, salt, and pepper.
- Spread on a baking sheet and roast for 25-30 minutes, until soft.
- Meanwhile, rinse the quinoa with cool water.
- Heat vegetable broth in a saucepan until it boils.
- Add the quinoa, decrease the heat to low, cover, and simmer for 15 minutes.
- Fluff the quinoa with a fork and serve with the roasted eggplant on top.

Nutritional Information: 320 calories, 10g fat, 50g carbs, 8g protein, low purines.

<u>Tofu and Broccoli Stir-fry</u>

- **Servings: two.**
- **Prep time: 15 minutes.**
- **Cooking Time: 10 minutes.**

Ingredients:

- One block of firm tofu, drained and cubed
- Two cups broccoli florets.
- One tablespoon of soy sauce.
- One tablespoon of sesame oil.
- One garlic clove, minced

Instructions:

- Press the tofu to remove extra moisture, then cut into cubes.
- Heat the sesame oil in a pan over medium heat.
- Cook garlic and tofu till golden brown.
- Add the broccoli and stir-fry until soft and crispy.
- Drizzle with soy sauce and toss until evenly coated.
- Serve hot.

Nutritional Information: 250 calories, 14g fat, 12g carbs, 20g protein, and low purines.

<u>Garlic Shrimp with Rice</u>

- **Servings: two.**
- **Prep time: 10 minutes.**
- **Cook time: 20 minutes.**

Ingredients:

- 8-ounce peeled and deveined shrimp
- One cup of cooked brown rice.
- 2 garlic cloves, minced
- One tablespoon of olive oil.
- Juice from 1 lemon
- Add salt and pepper to taste.

Instructions:

- Heat the olive oil in a skillet over medium heat.
- Add the garlic and heat until fragrant.
- Add the shrimp and cook until pink and opaque.
- Squeeze lemon juice over the shrimp and season with salt and pepper.
- Serve on a bed of brown rice.

Nutritional Information: 300 calories, 8g fat, 30g carbs, 25g protein, low purines.

<u>Beefless Stew</u>

- **Servings: four.**
- **Prep time: 15 minutes.**
- **Cooking Time: 40 minutes.**

Ingredients:

- 2 cups of meatless beef pieces or seitan
- Four cups of veggie broth.
- Two potatoes, diced
- Two carrots, sliced
- 1 onion, chopped
- Two tablespoons of tomato paste.
- One teaspoon thyme.
- Add salt and pepper to taste.

Instructions:

- In a large pot, sauté the onions until transparent.
- Combine the beefless beef chunks, potatoes, carrots, and vegetable broth.
- Stir in the tomato paste and thyme.
- Bring to a boil, then reduce and simmer for 30-40 minutes.
- Season with salt and pepper.
- Serve hot.

Nutritional Information: 250 calories, 2g fat, 45g carbs, 15g protein, low purines.

Spaghetti Squash Primavera

- **Servings: two.**
- **Prep time: 10 minutes.**
- **Cook for 45 minutes.**

Ingredients:

- One spaghetti squash, halved and seeded
- One cup cherry tomato, halved
- 1 zucchini, sliced
- 1 bell pepper, sliced
- Two teaspoons of olive oil.
- One teaspoon of Italian seasoning.
- Add salt and pepper to taste.

Instructions:

- Preheat the oven to 400°F (200° C). Km
- Drizzle the spaghetti squash halves with olive oil, salt, and pepper.
- Place the cut side down on a baking sheet and roast for 40 minutes.
- In a pan, cook tomatoes, zucchini, and bell pepper with Italian spice.
- With a fork, scrape the squash into strands.
- Combine the veggie mixture with the spaghetti squash strands.
- Serve warm.

Nutritional Information: 180 calories, 7g fat, 30g carbs, 3g protein, low purines.

<u>Cherry Tomato Bruschetta.</u>

- **Servings: four.**
- **Prep time: 10 minutes.**
- **Cook for 5 minutes.**

Ingredients:

- 2 cups cherry tomatoes, halved
- 1/4 cup of fresh basil, chopped
- 2 garlic cloves, minced
- One tablespoon of balsamic vinegar.
- One tablespoon of olive oil.
- Add salt and pepper to taste.
- 4 slices of whole grain baguette, toasted

Instructions:

- In a bowl, combine the tomatoes, basil, garlic, balsamic vinegar, and olive oil.
- Season with salt and pepper.
- Spoon the mixture onto the toasted baguette slices.
- Serve immediately.

Nutritional Information: 150 calories, 5g fat, 20g carbs, 5g protein, low purines.

Cauliflower Buffalo Bites

- **Servings: four.**
- **Prep time: 10 minutes.**
- **Cook time: 20 minutes.**

Ingredients:

- Four cups cauliflower florets.
- 1/2 cup Buffalo sauce.
- One tablespoon of olive oil.

Instructions:

- Preheat the oven to 450°F (230° C).
- Combine cauliflower florets, olive oil, and buffalo sauce.
- Spread onto a baking sheet and roast for 20 minutes.
- Serve hot with a side of gout-friendly ranch dressing.

Nutritional Information: 100 calories, 7g fat, 8g carbs, 2g protein, and low purines.

<u>Zucchini Chips</u>

- **Servings: two.**
- **Prep time: 10 minutes.**
- **Cooking Time: 2 hours.**

Ingredients:

- Two thinly sliced zucchinis
- One tablespoon of olive oil.
- Salt to taste.

Instructions:

- Preheat the oven to 225°F (105° C).
- Toss the zucchini slices with olive oil and salt.
- Arrange the slices in a single layer on a baking sheet.
- Bake for two hours, or until crisp.
- Let cool before serving.

Nutritional Information: 100 calories, 7g fat, 8g carbs, 2g protein, and low purines.

<u>**Watermelon Salad**</u>

- **Servings: four.**
- **Prep time: 15 minutes.**

Ingredients:

- 4 cups watermelon, diced
- 1/2 cup crumbled feta cheese.
- 1/4 cup fresh mint, chopped
- Two teaspoons of olive oil.
- Juice from 1 lime

Instructions:

- In a large bowl, combine the watermelon, feta cheese, and mint.
- Drizzle with olive oil and lime juice.
- Gently toss to blend.
- Serve cold.

Nutritional Information: 180 calories, 9g fat, 22g carbs, 5g protein, low purines.

<u>Cottage Cheese with Pineapple</u>

- **Servings: two.**
- **Prep time: 5 minutes.**

Ingredients:

- One cup of low-fat cottage cheese
- 1 cup diced pineapple.

Instructions:

- Divide the cottage cheese into two bowls.
- Garnish with diced pineapple.
- Serve immediately, or refrigerate before serving.

Nutritional Information: 180 calories, 2g fat, 20g carbs, 20g protein, low purines.

<u>Roasted Chickpeas.</u>

- **Servings: four.**
- **Prep time: 5 minutes.**
- **Cook for 30-40 minutes.**

Ingredients:

- 1 can (15 oz) of drained and rinsed chickpeas
- One tablespoon of olive oil.
- 1/2 teaspoons smoked paprika.
- Salt to taste.

Instructions:

- Preheat your oven to 400°F (200°C).
- Dry the chickpeas with paper towels.
- Toss the chickpeas with olive oil, smoked paprika, and salt.
- Arrange on a baking sheet in a single layer.
- Roast for 30-40 minutes, stirring the pan occasionally, or until crisp.
- Let cool before serving.

Nutritional Information: 120 calories, 4g fat, 18g carbs, 6g protein, low purines.

<u>Stuffed Mushrooms</u>

- **Servings: four.**
- **Prep time: 15 minutes.**
- **Cook time: 20 minutes.**

Ingredients:

- 16 entire white mushrooms with stems removed.
- 1/2 cup of low-fat cream cheese
- 1/4 cup grated parmesan cheese.
- 1/4 cup of minced parsley.
- 2 garlic cloves, minced
- Add salt and pepper to taste.

Instructions:

- Preheat the oven to 350°F/175°C.
- In a bowl, combine the cream cheese, Parmesan, parsley, and garlic.
- Season with salt and pepper.
- Fill the mushroom caps with the mixture.
- Transfer to a baking sheet and bake for 20 minutes.
- Serve warm.

Nutritional Information: 100 calories, 6g fat, 4g carbs, 8g protein, and low purines.

<u>**Sweet Potato Fries**</u>

- **Servings: four.**
- **Prep time: 10 minutes.**
- **Cook for 25-30 minutes.**

Ingredients:

- Peel two large sweet potatoes and chop them into fries.
- Two teaspoons of olive oil.
- 1/2 teaspoon paprika.
- Salt to taste.

Instructions:

- Preheat your oven to 425°F (220°C).
- Combine sweet potato fries, olive oil, paprika, and salt.
- Arrange in a single layer on a baking sheet.
- Bake for 25-30 minutes, rotating once, or until crisp.
- Serve hot.

Nutritional Information: 150 calories, 7g fat, 20g carbs, 2g protein, low purines.

<u>Kale Chips</u>

- **Servings: two.**
- **Prep time: 5 minutes.**
- **Cook for 10-15 minutes.**

Ingredients:

- One bunch of kale, stems trimmed and leaves torn.
- One tablespoon of olive oil.
- Salt to taste.

Instructions:

- Preheat the oven to 350°F/175°C.
- Combine kale leaves, olive oil, and salt.
- Arrange on a baking sheet in a single layer.
- Bake for 10-15 minutes, until the edges are crispy but not browned.
- Let cool before serving.

Nutritional Information: 80 calories, 7g fat, 5g carbs, 2g protein, low purines.

<u>Fruit Kabobs</u>

- **Servings: four.**
- **Prep time: 10 minutes.**

Ingredients:

- 1 cup strawberries, halved
- 1 cup cubed cantaloupe.
- 1 cup pineapple, cubed
- One cup of grapes
- Four wooden skewers.

Instructions:

- Thread strawberries, cantaloupe, pineapple, and grapes on skewers.
- Arrange the fruit kabobs on a dish.
- Serve immediately or chill until ready to serve.

Nutritional Information: 90 calories, 0.5g fat, 22g carbs, 1g protein, and low purines.

Baked Apples with Cinnamon.

- **Servings: two.**
- **Prep time: 10 minutes.**
- **Cook for 30 minutes.**

Ingredients:

- Two big, cored apples
- Two teaspoons of cinnamon.
- One teaspoon of honey (optional)
- One-quarter cup water

Instructions:

• Preheat the oven to 350°F/175°C.

• Arrange the apples in a baking dish and sprinkle with cinnamon.

• Drizzle with honey if desired.

• Pour water into the bottom of the dish.

• Bake for 30 minutes, or until the apples are soft.

Nutritional Information: 95 calories, 0.3g fat, 25g carbs, 0.5g protein, and low purines.

<u>Pineapple Sorbet</u>

- **Servings: four.**
- **Preparation time: 5 minutes (including freezing time)**

Ingredients:

- Four cups frozen pineapple chunks.
- One tablespoon of honey (optional)
- Juice from 1 lime

Instructions:

- Combine frozen pineapple, honey (if using), and lime juice in a blender.
- Blend until smooth, scraping the sides as necessary.
- Transfer to a container and freeze until firm, about 2 hours.
- Scoop and serve.

Nutritional Information: 120 calories, 0.2g fat, 32g carbs, 1g protein, and low purines.

<u>Carrot Cake Muffins</u>

- **Serves: 12**
- **Prep time: 15 minutes.**
- **Cook time: 20 minutes.**

Ingredients:

- 1 1/2 cup whole wheat flour.
- One teaspoon of baking soda.
- 1/4 teaspoon of salt.
- One teaspoon of ground cinnamon.
- 1/2 cup unsweetened applesauce.
- One-quarter cup honey
- 1 egg
- One teaspoon of vanilla extract.
- One cup shredded carrot.
- 1/4 cup of chopped walnuts (optional).

Instructions:

- Preheat the oven to 350°F/175°C and line a muffin tray with paper liners.
- In a bowl, combine the flour, baking soda, salt, and cinnamon.
- In another bowl, combine the applesauce, honey, egg, and vanilla.
- Mix wet and dry ingredients until just combined.
- Fold in the carrots and walnuts, if using.
- Divide the batter among the muffin cups.
- Bake for 20 minutes, or until a toothpick comes out clean.

Nutritional Information: 110 calories, 1g fat, 24g carbs, 3g protein, low purines.

<u>Strawberry Gelatine</u>

- **Servings: four.**
- **Preparation time: 10 minutes, plus chilling time.**
- **Cook for 5 minutes.**

Ingredients:

- 2 cups fresh, hulled strawberries
- One cup of water.
- One tablespoon of gelatin powder.
- One tablespoon of honey (optional)

Instructions:

- Puree the strawberries in a blender until smooth.
- In a saucepan, sprinkle gelatine over water and set aside for a few minutes.
- Heat gently until the gelatine dissolves, then whisk in the strawberry puree and honey, if desired.
- Pour into Molds or a dish, then chill for about 2 hours.

Nutritional Information: 50 calories, 0.4g fat, 11g carbs, 2g protein, low purines.

<u>Banana Ice Cream.</u>

- **Servings: two.**
- **Preparation time: 5 minutes (including freezing time)**

Ingredients:

- Two ripe bananas cut and frozen

Instructions:

- Put frozen banana slices into a food processor or blender.
- Blend until smooth, scraping the sides as necessary.
- Serve immediately for soft-serve consistency, or freeze for another hour for firmer ice cream.

Nutritional Information: 105 calories, 0.3g fat, 27g carbs, 1.3g protein, low purines.

<u>**Pumpkin Pie Pudding**</u>

- **Servings: four.**
- **Prep time: 10 minutes.**

Ingredients:

- 1 can (15 oz) of pumpkin puree
- 1 1/2 cups low-fat or almond milk.
- 1/4 cup maple syrup.
- 2 tablespoons of pumpkin pie spice.
- 1/4 cup cornstarch.

Instructions:

- In a saucepan, combine the pumpkin puree, milk, maple syrup, pumpkin pie spice, and cornstarch.
- Cook over medium heat, stirring continuously, until the mixture thickens.
- Pour into serving dishes and refrigerate for at least two hours.

Nutritional Information: 140 calories, 1g fat, 30g carbs, 3g protein, low purines.

<u>Coconut Rice Pudding</u>

- **Servings: four.**
- **Prep time: 5 minutes.**
- **Cook time: 25 minutes.**

Ingredients:

- One cup of cooked white rice.
- One can (14 ounces) coconut milk
- One-quarter cup sugar
- 1/2 teaspoon of vanilla extract.

Instructions:

- In a saucepan, mix cooked rice, coconut milk, and sugar.
- Cook over medium heat for about 25 minutes, stirring periodically, until thickened.
- Remove from heat and mix in the vanilla extract.
- Serve either warm or cooled.

Nutritional Information: 260 calories, 14g fat, 34g carbs, 3g protein, and low purines.

<u>Peach Crisp</u>

- **Servings: six.**
- **Prep time: 15 minutes.**
- **Cook for 30 minutes.**

Ingredients:

- Four cups sliced peaches.
- 1/2 cup rolled oats.
- One-quarter cup almond flour
- One-quarter cup brown sugar
- 1/4 cup unsalted butter melted
- One-half teaspoon cinnamon

Instructions:

- Preheat your oven to 375°F (190°C).
- Place the peaches in a baking dish.
- In a bowl, combine the oats, almond flour, brown sugar, melted butter, and cinnamon until crumbly.
- Sprinkle the oat mixture over the peaches.
- Bake for 30 minutes, or until the top is golden brown.

Nutritional Information: 180 calories, 8g fat, 27g carbs, 3g protein, low purines.

<u>Chocolate Avocado Mousse.</u>

- **Servings: two.**
- **Prep time: 10 minutes.**

Ingredients:

- One ripe avocado.
- 1/4 cup cocoa powder.
- 1/4 cup honey or maple syrup.
- 1/2 teaspoon of vanilla extract.
- A pinch of salt.

Instructions:

- Transfer the avocado flesh to a blender.
- Combine the cocoa powder, honey, vanilla extract, and salt.
- Blend until smooth.
- Divide among serving dishes and refrigerate before serving.

Nutritional Information: 320 calories, 15g fat, 50g carbs, 4g protein, low purines.

<u>Lemon Bars</u>

- **Serves: 8**
- **Prep time: 15 minutes.**
- **Cook time: 35 minutes.**

Ingredients:

For the crust:

- One cup of almond flour.
- 1/4 cup melted coconut oil.
- One spoonful of honey.

For the Filling:

- 3 eggs
- One-half cup honey
- 1/2 cup of lemon juice.
- Two tablespoons of almond flour.

Instructions:

- Preheat the oven to 350°F/175°C.
- Combine almond flour, coconut oil, and honey for the crust, then press it into the bottom of a buttered 8x8-inch pan.
- Bake 15 minutes, or until slightly brown.
- To make the filling, whisk together eggs, honey, lemon juice, and almond flour.
- Pour over the baked crust, then return to the oven.
- Bake for 20 minutes, or until the filling has set.
- Let cool completely before cutting into bars.

Nutritional Information: calories: 230, fat: 14g, carbs: 24g, protein: 6g, purines: low.

CHAPTER 8: LIVING WELL WITH GOUT.

Exercise and Gout: Senior-Safe Activities.

Exercise is a crucial part of controlling gout, particularly for seniors. While high-impact activities may not be appropriate, there are numerous low-impact exercises that can promote joint health and overall well-being without increasing gout symptoms.

Walking

Walking is a low-impact activity that is easy to add into one's everyday routine. It improves cardiovascular health and can be adjusted to suit individual comfort levels.

Swimming and water aerobics

Swimming and water aerobics are great exercises for persons who have gout. Water's buoyancy minimizes joint stress, making it a more comfortable approach to workout.

Cycling

Stationary cycling and outdoor biking are excellent choices for low-impact cardiovascular exercise. They allow for joint movement without the high impact found in other forms of training.

Yoga & Pilates

Yoga and Pilates can increase flexibility, strength, and balance while being easy on the joints. They may be adjusted to your comfort level and are good for stress relief.

Tai Chi

Tai Chi is a martial technique that emphasizes slow, deliberate motions and deep breathing. It is believed to improve balance and reduce stress, both of which are beneficial for gout treatment.

Low-impact sports.

Low-impact activities such as golf or bowling can be entertaining and provide moderate exercise without putting excessive strain on the joints.

Tips for Exercise with Gout:

- Listen to Your Body: If you experience pain or discomfort, take a break or switch to a different activity.
- Stay Hydrated: Drink plenty of water before, during, and after exercise to help your body eliminate uric acid.
- Warm-Up and Cool-Down: Begin with mild stretching to prepare your body for exercise, then cool down to reduce muscle stiffness.
- Wear Proper Footwear: To preserve your joints, choose shoes with adequate support and cushioning.
- Consult Your Doctor: Before beginning any new fitness plan, speak with your doctor, especially if you have gout.

During a gout flare-up, it is advised to rest the affected joint and avoid exertion until the inflammation has subsided. Using ice and taking prescribed medicine can assist to alleviate symptoms at this time. Once the flare-up has subsided, you can gradually resume your exercise regimen, focusing on low-impact exercises to stay active and healthy.

CHAPTER 9: BONUS.

Gout-Friendly Foods List

Fruits

- Cherries may help reduce the frequency of gout attacks.
- Citrus fruits, such as oranges and lemons, have low purine content.
- Berries: Strawberries, blueberries, and raspberries are gout-friendly fruits.
- Apples are a good low-purine snack.
- Pineapple: Known for its anti-inflammatory properties.

Vegetables

- Leafy greens: Such as lettuce, spinach, and kale.
- Cruciferous vegetables: Including broccoli, cauliflower, and cabbage.
- Root vegetables: Carrots, beets, and turnips are safe options.
- Squash, both summer and winter types.
- Potatoes: Can be consumed in moderation.

Proteins

- Eggs: A flexible protein source with minimal purine content.
- Legumes: Beans, lentils, and peas are good plant-based protein sources.
- Low-fat dairy: Such as milk, yogurt, and cheese, which may help lower uric acid levels.
- Tofu: A soy-based protein that's a viable alternative to meat.

Grains

- Whole grains like oats, brown rice, and barley are recommended.
- Quinoa: A nutrient-rich seed that's a good alternative to high-purine grains.

Nuts and Seeds

- Almonds and walnuts: In moderation, as they give healthful fats.
- Flaxseeds and chia seeds: Rich in omega-3 fatty acids.

Beverages

• Water is required for the body to eliminate uric acid.

• Tea and coffee can be consumed in moderation.

Fat and Oils

- Olive oil: A nutritious fat that promotes general wellness.
- Avocado oil is another excellent source of monounsaturated fats.

Herbs and spices

- Turmeric and ginger are known for their anti-inflammatory properties.
- Basil, rosemary, and thyme can provide taste without introducing purines.

Others

- Consume low-purine fish such as salmon in moderation.
- Whole-grain products: Look for whole-grain stamps or components that say "whole wheat flour".

It's crucial to remember that, while these foods are generally acceptable for gout sufferers, individual tolerances may differ. Seniors should evaluate their reactions to various meals and modify their diet accordingly.

Additionally, keeping a healthy weight and staying hydrated are critical components of gout management. Always get customized dietary guidance from a healthcare professional or a licensed dietitian.

14-Day Meal Plan

Day 1:

- Breakfast is Sunny Citrus Parfait.
- Lunch is Quinoa Tabbouleh.
- Dinner: baked salmon with dill.
- Snack: Cherry tomato bruschetta.
- Dessert: Baked apples with cinnamon.

Day 2:

- Breakfast: cherry oatmeal delight.
- Lunch: Grilled chicken salad.
- Dinner: Stuffed bell peppers.
- Snack: Cauliflower Buffalo Bites.
- Dessert: pineapple sorbet.

Day 3:

- Breakfast: Egg-White Vegetable Scramble.
- Lunch: Lentil soup with vegetables.
- Dinner: grilled turkey burgers.
- Snack: Zucchini chips.
- Dessert: Carrot Cake Muffins.

Day 4:

- Breakfast: Almond butter toast.
- Lunch: Turkey and Avocado Wrap.
- Dinner: Vegetable lasagna
- Snack: Watermelon salad.
- Dessert: strawberry gelatine.

Day 5:

- Breakfast: Berry-banana smoothie.
- Lunch: Cucumber sandwiches.
- Dinner: Lemon-Herb Chicken
- Snack: Cottage cheese with pineapple.
- Dessert: banana ice cream.

Day 6:

- Breakfast: Apple Cinnamon Porridge.
- Lunch: Carrot and Ginger Puree.
- Dinner: Roasted eggplant with quinoa.
- Snack: roasted chickpeas.
- Dessert is Pumpkin Pie Pudding.

Day 7:

- Breakfast: tomato basil omelette.
- Lunch: Tofu Stir-Fry.
- Dinner: Tofu and Broccoli Stir-Fry
- Snack: Stuffed mushrooms.
- Dessert: coconut rice pudding.

Day 8:

- Breakfast: Avocado Egg Salad.
- Lunch: Mediterranean chickpea salad.
- Dinner: Garlic shrimp with rice.
- Snack: Sweet Potato fries.
- Dessert: peach crisp.

Day 9:

- Breakfast - Peachy Keen Muesli
- Lunch: Pumpkin soup.
- Dinner: Beefless stew.
- Snack: Kale chips.
- Dessert is Chocolate Avocado Mousse.

Day 10:

- Breakfast - Spinach and Feta Wrap
- Lunch: Broccoli with Pine Nut Pasta
- Dinner: Spaghetti squash primavera.
- Snack: Fruit Kebabs
- Dessert: Lemon bars.

Day 11:

- Breakfast is Sunny Citrus Parfait.
- Lunch is Quinoa Tabbouleh.
- Dinner: baked salmon with dill.
- Snack: Cherry tomato bruschetta.
- Dessert: Baked apples with cinnamon.

Day 12:

- Breakfast: cherry oatmeal delight.
- Lunch: Grilled chicken salad.
- Dinner: Stuffed bell peppers.
- Snack: Cauliflower Buffalo Bites.
- Dessert: pineapple sorbet.

Day 13:

- Breakfast: Egg-White Vegetable Scramble.
- Lunch: Lentil soup with vegetables.
- Dinner: grilled turkey burgers.
- Snack: Zucchini chips.
- Dessert: Carrot Cake Muffins.

Day 14:

- Breakfast: Almond butter toast.
- Lunch: Turkey and Avocado Wrap.
- Dinner: Vegetable lasagna
- Snack: Watermelon salad.
- Dessert: strawberry gelatine.

CONCLUSION

As we conclude this culinary journey, I hope that "Gout Diet Cookbook for Seniors" has offered you with not just a collection of tasty recipes, but also a fresh viewpoint on managing gout through nutrition. The recipes we've given are intended to bring joy to your table while also keeping your health in mind. Each dish has been carefully prepared to be low in purines while great in flavor.

Remember that controlling gout involves more than just avoiding certain foods; it also entails adopting a lifestyle that includes balanced nutrition, frequent exercise, and awareness. This cookbook seeks to be a companion on that journey, providing instruction and inspiration with each recipe.

I welcome you to try these dishes, play around with Flavors, and make each meal a celebration of health and enjoyment. And as you do, I'd appreciate it if you could share your experiences. Your comment is invaluable—it not only assists others in their search for a gout-friendly diet, but it also contributes to the ever-expanding community of health-conscious people.

If you loved this cookbook, please consider giving it a favorable review on Amazon. Honest reviews educate others on the benefits of a gout-friendly diet and provide valuable feedback for future editions. Your help is much appreciated.

Thank you for choosing this cookbook, and may your meals be as satisfying as they are delicious. Wishing you good health and joy!